F.I.T.
(Finding Increments of Time)
Journal

By *KIMBERLY "KIMMY" ROSS*

F.I.T.
(Finding Increments of Time)
Journal

Kimberly Ross

ISBN-13:978-1544980416
ISBN-10-1544980418

Kimmy F.I.T. Fitness, LLC
11600 Shadow Creek Pkwy #111, #136
Pearland, TX 77584
kimmyfitfitness@gmail.com

Book cover designs by Brittney Molina
Photos by Troy Thomas (El Grande PapiRatzi)
Interior formatting by Polgarus Studio

Published by
Kimmy F.I.T. Fitness, LLC, Pearland, TX

Printed in the United States of America

"When you limit yourself by what you are not willing to do, you limit yourself from what you CAN do."

PREFACE

Can we just be honest? Health, wellness, and fitness have gotten quite complicated these days. The health and wellness industry is a multi-billion dollar industry. There is a tremendous amount of information to sort through with very few user-friendly approaches to making any sense of it all. Have you ever visited a nice restaurant that had a vast array of menu options? I mean, the menu had like four pages of options. You thought, "Wow this is great!" The reality is, after asking your server to come back multiple times, you remained undecided and defaulted to your same old selections. It may not necessarily be a healthy selection, but it is the selection that is familiar to you.

They say, "a confused mind does nothing". Doing nothing or defaulting to bad choices is sort of what has landed most of the American population where it is today: in a state of poor health — obesity, diabetes, hypertension, and stress to pinpoint a few.

As a Registered Nurse who has spent much of her career caring for patients with chronic illnesses, and as a Pharmaceutical Sales Representative selling prescription medications, I became keenly aware of our misuse of healthcare resources, primarily due to the misuse of our God-given bodies.

I then decided to create this journal to serve a real purpose for you. I am "old school" in the sense that I like to write things down on paper with a pen. When it comes to documenting things, I prefer pen and paper over computers and emails. I remember when nursing documentation transitioned over to electronic medical records, it was a huge adjustment to my way of working. I despised the thought of it. To me, it was like creating a disconnect between my voice (as the patient's advocate) and the care I was providing. Yes, since that time, I have adapted to the current means of communication (excessive text messages and emails); however, there is something about putting pen to paper and seeing words come to life.

That is how I thought this journal could serve you. Within the covers of this book, I want to create a space for you to have small "pep talks" with yourself. I want you to be able to be honest on these pages about the plans and commitments you are willing to keep as you journey towards a more fit lifestyle. In this journal, you will be assigned tasks and I will challenge you to do a few things that you may not be comfortable with. Let's just be upfront about that now. I believe that as we are faithful in the little things, we also prepare and position ourselves to have faith in and receive bigger things. So, even if you are unsure if you completely trust me just yet, if you are willing to trust the *process,* you will find value in this journal.

As I mentioned earlier, things have gotten complex. Many people think this "fitness thing" is 100% exercising all the time while counting every macro and micronutrient that goes into yours and your family's meals. It is not. Realistically, life is too busy for the typical person to be spending countless hours in a gym, recreational facility, or in their kitchen.

My desire is to provide the tools, tips, and resources that you will not find in this capacity anywhere else. I will help simplify your life in the areas of health, wellness, and fitness.

Here is your first **FREE Bonus**:

If you acknowledge that your nutritional habits are a part of your lack luster physical results, you are more than likely 100% correct. In the fitness world, it is said that *'results are 80% nutrition and 20% exercise'*.

When it comes to nutrition, one size does **NOT** fit all. With that being said, your FREE bonus is a confidential online health assessment based on your diet, lifestyle, body type, physical condition, health issues and medications. This revolutionary approach to vitamin supplementation is customized to your specific needs. This scientific assessment tool means no more guesswork for you. You will get personalized recommendations only for what you NEED. After completing the assessment, I am suggesting this agreement:

Try ID Life - Your commitment to yourself
Simplify your Life - My commitment to you

Assessment link: **www.whynottry.idlife.com**

You are unique.
Your nutrition should be too.

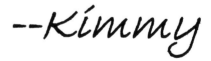

Contents

"Exercise is a celebration of what your body can do.
Not a punishment for what you ate."

INTRODUCTION

Regular physical exercise can be fun and it is essential to your health. In this *F.I.T. Journal*, I want to see people just like you become more and more active each day. This can occur over time with consistent and committed actions:

DAILY COMMITMENTS:

1. Use this journal (your promise)
2. Complete the daily input (be honest)
3. Implement realistic and sustainable behaviors (celebrate each success)

The older we get, the busier our lives become and the less time we make for an enjoyable exercise regimen.

If you have decided that you are ready to commit to **F.I.T.** (Finding Increments of Time), but you are not accustomed to physical activity or you have some health concerns that may need to be addressed first, I advise you to check with your healthcare provider before starting any exercise program. This is to ensure that you are ready to go!

If there are any health challenges present, it does not necessarily mean that you cannot start. You may be able to do any activity you want with slow and safe progression depending on your restriction(s).

WHO AM I?

Who am I? I am Kimberly Ross of *Kimmy F.I.T. Fitness, LLC*. I have been a Registered Nurse and a Nurse Educator for more than 20 years combined. I served in the United States Air Force teaching, training, implementing, and overseeing programs geared toward successful population health outcomes. While also serving as the squadron's fitness monitor for the 52nd Medical Operations, I became enthralled in instructional fitness and helping others reach their physical fitness goals. Later in life, I began teaching fitness, personal training, and competing in bodybuilding figure competitions. I earned my place in the professional bodybuilding arena. And, at present, I have earned 3 professional qualifications with three natural, drug-tested (drug-free) bodybuilding federations.

I am a native of Detroit, Michigan. I currently reside in a growing suburb of Houston, Texas with my dog, Diamond. The last several years of my nursing career have been spent as a Pharmaceutical Sales Representative and Nurse Educator. During this time, I was involved in prescription drug sales with well-known multi-million dollar companies. The money was good, but the rewards (other than materialistic tangibles) were subpar. The more enlightened I became about the impact of prescription drugs, their side effects and some of their strategies for bringing certain drugs to market, the more I struggled with my passion and purpose versus a paycheck.

Do not misunderstand me. I do believe that I supported a few of the "best" drugs on the market for all intent and purposes. I also realize what needs to happen: We as people need to stop depending completely on "Big Pharma" and our doctors for health care.

The health care that is available today should really be referred to as "sick" care. Seeking reactive and temporary fixes to our ailments in the form of excessive prescription medications that cause nutrient-depleting side effects and new symptoms, rather than addressing the underlying issue is not the answer. The focus needs to be on wellness and disease prevention, and it starts with us.

So why would a single, healthy woman who was making a great salary eventually become tarnished by the "golden ticket" known as a 6-figure corporate paycheck?

Well, I am glad you asked. See, my story is not one of "weight loss", nor do I believe that everyone else's fitness journey is a weight loss story. In fact, I was never physically fat, overweight, or obese. Do I sound perfect yet? Keep reading because I was "emotionally fat."

I grew up in Detroit as the only child of a single discontented mother and a distant, troubled father. My childhood was full of demands and responsibilities.

My mother struggled as a teen mom. She desired to have a normal teenage life but was held accountable for the responsibilities of her unplanned pregnancy. She had to grow up and come to terms with those feelings as well as her feelings of resentment, but I don't think she was ever able to reconcile it all. When my mother later married my stepfather, it was then that I began to struggle with loneliness.

I believe that loneliness, coupled with parents who lacked proper parenting skills, created a chain linked by rejection, depression, and self-doubt. I found myself longing for valuable and authentic relationships.

I needed to feel a part of something. I needed to feel included and loved. I sought inclusion via exclusive groups, sports, sororities, and church ministries. I sought after corporate jobs and esteemed positions within the military.

Those groups served their purpose to some degree, but I still felt I was never made to just fit in. I knew I was different and there was more I was meant to do and to be, but fitting into anyone's box was not it. Many years to follow would reveal a truer path. It is clear now that health and fitness have become my platform for purpose.

I recognized how the love and mastery of nursing enabled me to be a change agent in transforming and impacting lives, *'one body at a time'*. I began teaching fitness classes and providing personal training in conjunction with my corporate job. I later parlayed my nursing and fitness expertise as well as tons of professional corporate training into another entrepreneurial opportunity with a science-based health and wellness company.

Now, I am showing you and others in a way that only I can: How to move forward successfully in your fitness journey while setting goals that are specific, measurable, attainable, realistic, and time-sensitive (S.M.A.R.T.). These kinds of goals help you accomplish small sustainable wins over time.

My mission is to help others who *appear* to have it all together, as well as those who are trying to get it together, balance their mental and physical well-being through the release of "emotional fat" and physical fat while building health and "*wellth*".

HOW TO USE THIS JOURNAL

What is this?

I like to describe this *F.I.T. Journal* as the first steps to your physical freedom. There are no complicated, unrealistic processes or promises. No *'fat-at-night skinny-by-daylight'* diet fads here. I am vehemently opposed to those! Essentially, this journal was created with YOU in mind. To hold you accountable to yourself first and then serve as a simplified outline for better choices.

In the pages to follow you will have space to write out your

- Self-talk
- Small and Big Wins
- Challenges
- Changes
- Goals

You will hear me cheering for you throughout the journal and your journey, encouraging you to stay the course and trust the process.

Who is this for?

Let's be clear. Everything is not for everyone. Such is life! But if you have tried multiple weight loss attempts and miraculous magical jungle juices only to find yourself still wanting to dive into a bucket of KFC, you are not alone and you have NOT failed. You have simply learned what does not or has not successfully worked for you in the past.

Our bodies are constantly changing. The health and fitness world sometimes over complicate things. Now you have a chance to reconsider what your journey can look like with more commitment, accountability, visualization and support.

What can you expect?

First and foremost, you can expect to hold yourself accountable. In purchasing this journal, you have already taken a commendable first step. I thank you for your purchase, but more importantly, I praise you for your show of commitment.

In the *F.I.T. Journal,* you will find increments of time to "write the vision and make it plain" (*Bible, Habakkuk 2:2*). However, this journal will only work if you do. Do not give up before you see results and please do not blame your setbacks or shortcomings on this amazing journal or its adorable author. The truth is: you are going to have to get honest with yourself in this new process.

Use these tips to guide you:

1. Prepare to get real, real honest with yourself
2. Make a list of *supportive* friends who you will call when you feel the urge to binge or slack off
3. Replace your negative thoughts and emotional fat with empowering statements
4. Don't just think about it! Journal about it! Most importantly, be about it!
5. Acknowledge what is and what is not working
6. Plan your food and workouts
7. Seek inspiration beyond just motivation
8. Visualize your success (not just your size)

9. Get out of your comfort zone by facing your fears and trashing your excuses
10. Give praise for ALL your efforts and good work
    Inhale. Exhale and let's have FUN with this!

Whether you work with me directly or follow me on social media, I can be reached via www.kimmyfitfitness.com or on Facebook @KimmyFITFitness. You can also request to join my private Kimmy's Fitness Community (KFC) group via Facebook @KimmysKFC.

Support is available whenever you need it.

Fair Enough?

ACKNOWLEDGEMENTS

This journal was created from my passion and experiences. I am sharing with you much of what I have learned. These lessons have been put into practice throughout my time as a nurse, fitness instructor and trainer, bodybuilder, and entrepreneur in health and wellness. I am forever on a quest to impact and amplify the lives of those who are in the midst of their own physical health journey.

To Suzan Hart of *The Hart Zone*. You have been an incredible mentor. Point-blank...end of story. You have helped me to sort through my processes, feelings, and my evolution of leadership. It is very rare that I observe someone and feel compelled to be in their space. Every moment spent learning with you is the fuel that drives me forward. Your perspective, loving energy and truth gave me the confidence to know that the universe does hear me when I speak. And it's my responsibility to powerfully choose and to say the right stuff. Our time together has not been enough.

Thank you.

To my Detroit girls, Dorothea "Doddie" Mbote, Millicent Little-George, and Maria Johnson. You all were only a phone call and many text messages away. Thank you for caring enough about me and what I was creating to give me timely and honest feedback.

Thank you to my exceptionally generous and talented editors Deborah Ferdinand of Creative Consulting Services and Sade Kristyna

(@SadeKristyna on Instagram). You both sorted out the weeds and the truth so skillfully. I would not have made it through this arduous process without your supportive help and insight.

Lastly, to all of those I have worked with in some capacity via my different professional endeavors and personal growth. It is because of every patient, customer, client, and friendly follower that I found the courage to share this with you. Thank you to the leaders who have and are leading me along the way. In the words of my favorite musical genius, Prince, *"When you get the inner calling to do something and you know that you're being inspired by God, then you pretty much know you better answer that call or answer the consequences"* The Larry King Show, 1999.

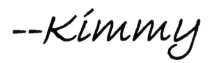

F.I.T.

(Finding Increments of Time)

Journal

By *KIMBERLY "KIMMY" ROSS*

CHAPTER 1
EMOTIONAL FAT

Webster's dictionary defines 'health' as being sound in body, mind, and spirit. Free from disease or pain.

I searched through *Webster's* entire listing of the letter "E" but I could not find "emotional fat". Let me tell you where I did find it.

Growing up most of my childhood as an only child, I frequently lost myself in encyclopedias, daydreaming, and long bike rides until the street lights came on. For 16 years, I was the only child to a single mother and a mostly distant father whom I loved and longed for dearly. Most of his life was spent often fighting his own demons. Under the authority of my mother and eventually my stepfather, my childhood was one of strict responsibilities, angst, and an obsessive imagination.

Like many of my friends, I was also a "latch-key kid". I would finish a day of schooling, walk or get bussed home, let myself inside with my house key, start my chores and homework, and wait with a bit of anxiety for my mother to come home from work. It was the expected routine in our household. Even more so when my stepfather entered our world. When we moved from my beloved grandmother's home, it seemed like it was my parents versus me. It was a difficult time of adjustment for me. My Nanny (maternal grandmother) was my guardian angel, my closest friend. I often found myself living in fear of death and dying. I almost obsessively worried about my Nanny now that there were miles between us after my mother and I moved away.

I feared her death. At the time, as far as I knew, she was healthy, but I had mini-panic attacks that no one knew about except her. I am sure she didn't have a name for it when I would call her freaking out on the phone while home alone worrying about her dying and leaving me alone with my parents. I didn't have a name for it either, but today, I'd like to think that I have a better understanding of it all.

When we talk about health and its mental component, emotions are worth noting. According to *Webster's*, emotions are defined as "conscious mental reactions experienced as strong feelings, accompanied by physiological and behavioral changes in the body" (*Webster's Online Dictionary*). Emotions affect the health of the body.

As a kid, I was being affected by the accumulation of what I have coined as "**emotional fat**." The mental heaviness of emotional fat weighed me down more than any physical weight ever has.

Have you not heard of emotional fat? Well, I could not find it in *Webster* or any other resource, but I had one of Oprah's *'Aha! moments'* when it came out of my mouth and onto the pages of this journal.

If we apply *Webster's* definition of emotions to the term "emotional fat", emotional fat can be stifling, stagnating and over-weighted thoughts that we carry in our minds on a constant daily basis. I describe this emotional fat as the "bad cholesterol" in our mind. It clogs (physiologically) our thoughts from fully internalizing our abilities, our sense of belonging, and our value. It can also cause us to suffer physically.

I recall getting headaches when my mother would pull into the driveway after work. The emotional fat linked to feeling overly criticized, not good enough, and excluded in our small triad of a family was very stressful. For me, the impact of emotional fat revealed itself mostly physiologically though it reared its deceiving head in my perception of my physical beauty as well.

Emotional fat is not necessarily the same as negative thinking. Negative thinking has garnished attention through the years with an overwhelming focus on positive thinking, as if doing one "fixes" the other.

In my opinion, it requires more than positive thinking and pixie dust to combat emotional fat. It requires us to use tools and incorporate habits that can be realistically used to release the weight of emotional fat. A few of my personal tools and habits are shared throughout this journal.

I am often asked how I, as a nurse begin my fitness and bodybuilding journey. I do not remember an exact moment in time as it relates to fitness per se; however, I do vividly recall my first conversation regarding body building.

I was always in the gym, and my workouts were often intense. On more than one occasion, I had been asked, "do you compete?" I laughed at the notion because, in my opinion, I was nowhere near physically or mentally prepared or interested in whatever that meant.

After a few insightful conversations with one particularly persistent woman, I decided to do some research and come to a decision.

I thought it would be a highly unlikely undertaking since I could not imagine making the dietary sacrifices. More specifically, the sacrifice of wine that I felt I needed in order to maintain my sanity in the pharmaceutical sales job I had at that time.

I decided to go to a prep camp as a spectator. You know, a friendly reconnaissance of sorts to see what all the hype was about, so maybe the lady who seemed to be recruiting me would leave me alone. I was clever enough to seat myself in the room so I could hear the male and female coaches giving instructions. I sat down, observed, jotted notes, and took pictures of women who I deemed were the ones to beat, should I decide to compete. There was one woman from the camp whose picture I stored on my phone. I looked at it often, along with others. Shortly thereafter, I purchased a VIP ticket and attended my very first bodybuilding show alone.

The first time I ever stepped on a stage to compete as a novice figure competitor was May 2012. I set a goal, made a plan, made the necessary sacrifices (including the wine), and took the plunge. My only goal was to NOT suck! I can only compare that experience to one of my all-time favorite movies, *ROCKY*.

The night of my very first show, I won 1st place in Masters (35 years old and older) and 2nd in place Open Short (all ages, 5'3" or shorter). Shortly after, I was rushed back behind the stage by the expeditors. I was so clueless wondering, '*Why do I have to go back? I already won.*' I was told I had to compete in the overall judging category.

As I stood on the stairs, prepared to return to the stage, I glanced up at the woman on the staircase in front of me—it was HER! The woman in the photo on my cell phone.I looked behind me to see if others were lining up with us. When I realized no one else was lining up, I literally thought they just picked me because they needed someone to be on stage with her. Well, essentially they did. They needed another top winner to face off against another top winner in the overall judging. I thought, surely, I was not good enough (hint: emotional fat) to "compete" against this woman! Well, I was wrong!

Our names were called, we walked on stage, posed, and awaited the results. I was having a ball! The time of my life! The announcer then said, *"The overall winner of the 2012 competition is first time competitor…"* I knew right at that moment it was me. Of course, I had already seen my opponent compete in a previous show. I could hear my small group of friends who had traveled to Galveston, Texas in their matching *"Team Kimmy"* t-shirts to support me screaming! Being totally and completely unfamiliar with bodybuilding etiquette (despite all the videos I had watched), I went immediately into what I now call the *"Jesus cry"*. I was so happy! It took only fifteen weeks, and I stepped in the proverbial boxing ring to compete against myself, my emotional fat, and my real-life Apollo Creed. An unknown competitor, an underdog named Kimmy took home three trophies that night and the title of Champ. It was my *ROCKY* scene come true!

Now, when I strut across the stage to pose in a sequined bikini and clear heels, I am confident that I will not suck. My goal will always be to shine in a way that reaches someone sitting in the audience (like I was years ago), on the verge of writing their own story.

The memory of that day still gives me chills.

My story continues to tell the tale of a young girl growing up, weighed down by emotional fat, feeling alone yet inspired by her own wild imagination and the tenacity to be somebody. I set out to prove I could do it. I am good enough despite the words spoken to me early on that were often contrary.

The premise of my story is not about any physical weight that I released. It's more about my ongoing struggle with emotional fat and the self-actualization that I have gained.

Physical Fat versus Emotional fat

1. Based on the definition given earlier, how would you describe your health?
2. In what way(s) does "emotional fat" resonate with you? Tweet me on Twitter @Blazze02 with the hashtag #emotionalfat.
3. What aspects of your health has hindered your fitness goals?

F.I.T. TIP:

The difference in you and your body this week versus next week depends on what you do during the next seven days to achieve your goals.

CHAPTER 2
BABY STEPS

The first week will consist of small fitness steps of faith to build your commitment. Consider these seven days as building blocks. Some days will require a bit more effort than others. Just as amino acids are the building blocks for muscles, your development over the course of the first week will be the building blocks for your healthy habits.

I completely understand that for many of you, this is a HUGE personal commitment. Although you may not remember the few dollars spent for this journal, I am confident that you will remember the time you will spend completing this journal. I am humbled by the mere thought of how it will touch and/or change a portion of your life in some small way.

You will be given increments of information that I have tried to break down into digestible parts. Each page builds upon the next so please use the first seven days to prepare for the upcoming thirty days.

If you know that you are challenged in the area of following through, and you find yourself procrastinating on the initial day-by-day processes, don't worry. Take as many days (within reason) as needed to do the things asked of you before moving on to the next assignment.

This journal will set you up for success.

Are you ready?

DAY 1

First thing in the morning, before coffee, tea or breakfast, get naked and take a good look at yourself in the mirror. That's right! I said *naked*. This is non-negotiable and it is where you begin taking inventory of your emotional fat. This is called 'mirror work', and it gives you a chance to reflect on yourself up close and personally.

Mirror work has allowed me to reflect on my image. I have often been asked, "have you always been skinny?". If you didn't know, most fitness professionals, especially bodybuilders, cringe at such a description. I often want to reply: *'Genetics don't push me out the door to go exercise or to pre-plan my meals'*. I also get asked, "Do you have children?", followed by, "Wait until you get to my age." I can only assume that I hear such rhetoric because people look at me and are searching for a way to understand their own emotional fat.

To answer the questions, no I have technically never had a problem with my weight. However, for many years and much like many individuals today, I would consider myself to have been "skinny fat". Skinny fat is a term used to describe women who appear somewhat in shape, although they can't do a push up. They may also have high-risk factors, poor eating habits, a muffin top (abdominal fat), abnormal metabolic lab results, and they may be part of those at-risk populations. Let's just say that I definitely did fit into a few of those categories.

No, I do not have children. However, I know many women who were overweight either before, during, and/or after childbirth. They have managed to attain and maintain an impressive state of health and wellness. Truly incredible.

As for my age, I am currently 45 years young and I am emboldened by the phrase, *"Age is mostly a matter of mind. If you don't mind, it doesn't matter.*" Naked self-reflection has given me the opportunity to sort through my thoughts, and I am confident it will be a beneficial tool on your journey.

MIRROR WORK

As you wake up, and begin your naked mirror work, and are standing in front of a mirror having a good look at yourself, look yourself in the eyes from head to toe. You must keep in mind that your analysis should be from a place of compassion and not criticism. We are our worse critics and we are rarely fair when it comes to judging ourselves. If we heard a friend talking about themselves the way we often view or speak of ourselves, we would reprimand them immediately; but somehow, it seems justifiable when we do it to ourselves.

Take a slow deep breath. Exhale and repeat it two more times. Take more time and more breaths if needed. It is all for good.

I want you to remain in this space for at least 30-45 seconds. Trust me; it may seem like an eternity in your naked vulnerable state. I am asking you to do this because, for some, this may feel extremely uncomfortable or downright weird. I encourage you to use this quiet space in time to become intimate with yourself.

As women, the only time we spend any considerable amount of time in the mirror is when we are getting ready, putting on cosmetic makeup, covering up our imperfections. As men, I suspect your time in the mirror is spent shaving or flexing — neither having much to do with real or deep introspection.

After 45 seconds, if any self-limiting, emotionally fat thoughts pass through your mind as it relates to what you are seeing in the mirror, write them down. This is not a free pass to beat up on yourself. So, limit it to 3 thoughts for now. Remain bravely NAKED! Keep your pen or pencil and this journal nearby.

Make eye contact with yourself again. When you are done, look at that same list you just created. If you have written any self-doubting or emotionally fat thoughts, I want you to cross them out one by one and rewrite a self-empowerment statement. I don't care if you don't fully believe it at this point. Fake it or faith it, until you make it. You will get there.

Examples

Emotional fat:
"I look like my dad. He was fat so I will likely just be fat."

Empowerment:
"I love that I resemble my dad, but I also love myself enough to take better care of my body. I am responsible for what I see in this mirror, not him."

I would love to hear about your release of emotional fat via the Mirror Work exercise.

Tweet me @Blazze02 using the hashtag #EmotionalFat.

DAY 1 - FIRST STEPS

1. Write out your "emotional fat" mirror work

1._____

2 _____

3 _____

2. Re-write your empowerment statement(s)

1 _____

2 _____

3 _____

3. How did the Mirror Work make you feel during and after the exercise?

1 _____

2 _____

3 _____

F.I.T. TIP:

Send yourself and your body a little love and gratitude each day. The more love you give to yourself, the more gratitude will follow. The more you fill your spirit with gratitude, the more you will value your health.

DAY 2

Repeat your new empowerment statements from Day 1. We can keep working from those, but feel free to add new ones as new doubts arise that try to derail you. In addition to the *F.I.T. Journal*, you may want to write your empowerment statements directly on your mirror or transcribe them on sticky notes where you are likely to see them and be reminded throughout the day. When you join *Kimmy's KFC* on Facebook, I welcome you to share them there.

Next, take some *before pictures*. You do not have to share them with anyone. If you choose to share them, feel free to edit or crop the photo to remove your facial identity. I have clients who make tons of excuses when it comes to taking progress pictures, but you'll see tons of selfies all over their social media pages. Ironic? Not really. What I am asking of you requires a bit of transparency. Most people become resistant amid transparency and vulnerability.

You do not need a fancy camera crew or anyone to assist you. You can do it yourself privately by setting up your phone using the countdown self-timer setting or simply by recording video. Make the recording and then replay the video, taking screen shots.

I suggest 3 body pictures wearing shorts and a sports bra (if a woman) facing forward, two side-facing poses with arms extended out in front of the body and a photo facing backwards. Stand in a tall upright position and preferably against an uncluttered wall. Once you have identified your photo area and set up, it becomes a no-brainer for future shoots. Save those pictures to your phone, or print them.

**It should be noted that the same outfit or similar should be worn for all photos. This makes it easier to compare between photos…That is until those clothing items become just too darn big. I'm claiming it for you!

DAY 2 - FIRST STEPS

1. What excuses, if any, did you use to put off taking your first set of pictures? Be honest.

1 _____

2 _____

3 _____

2. What were your thoughts after you took the pictures?

1 _____

2 _____

3 _____

3. write down a few positive self image statements (I can, I am, I feel, I see). Right here. Right now. I'll wait...

1 _____

2 _____

3 _____

F.I.T. TIP:

There is a lot going on with you. Do not try to tackle it all at once. Pinpoint what is hindering you most at this moment. Be specific and attack it with vigor.

DAY 3

Today is important. You may want to grab a cup of green tea. I am going to ask you to identify your *WHY?* As you begin to move forward and towards better health, I ask that you look beyond class reunions, family vacations, or running into an ex-lover (though I must admit that this one does yield some motivation...just sayin').

Some of us find ourselves trying to keep up with the Joneses and we don't even know them. If we do know them, we probably don't like them, as we are too busy trying to measure up to them. As the popular quote goes, "you spend money you don't have to buy things you don't need to try and impress people you don't even like".

We have been led to believe in going hard, going fast, and to keep going to the point of exhaustion and burnout. I am asking you what do you wish to accomplish? What is different NOW compared to three or six months ago? What has changed in your life that has caused you to pick up this book?

Women specifically are the masters of self-sacrifice. God has blessed us with the ability to do things that men innately cannot do as effectively. Truthfully, women are the foundation of the world. Our ancestors were the backbone of families, communities, and movements.
We birth life to other human beings while risking our own lives in doing so, and then we commit our lives to raising those little humans

into adulthood. We are often the masterminds and support systems behind many great things, regularly investing our time, energy, and resources into things we deem valuable.

Where do *YOU* fit in all of this?

DAY 3 - FIRST STEPS

1. What is your WHY?

1 _____

2 _____

3 _____

2. How will you begin to put yourself first or as a higher priority?

1 _____

2 _____

3 _____

F.I.T. TIP:

Decide firmly in advance what you are committed to accomplishing. This holds you accountable and more likely to follow through.

DAY 4

Identify your Support. Who is likely to be your pusher? Who will be your voice of reason? Who or what is your Inspiration? Identify your team. By the way, count me in!

Now, listen. There will be days when you feel like this is the road less traveled. That's because it is. If it was super easy, everyone would be at their "goal weight," and the healthiest version of their self. If it was so easy to do it alone, your friends wouldn't need this journal and you would not need to tell everyone about it (see what I did there?). It does get tough. So, help by sharing this journal with them.

DAY 4 - FIRST STEPS

1. List your F.I.T. FIVE (5) supporters and their phone numbers. People who will keep you encouraged and accountable when you feel like binging or quitting.

1 _____

2 _____

3 _____

4 _____

5 _____

6. BONUS #2: KimmyFITFitness@gmail.com

2. If I had a magic wand, what 2 areas of your personal health or physical body would you want to improve?

1 _____

2 _____

F.I.T. TIP:

"If you want to go fast, go alone. If you want to go far, go with someone."
- African Proverb

DAY 5

Have you noticed the pace of this process thus far? I am confident that baby steps are a great approach to tackling health and fitness goals. We already agree that there is way too much to try to sort through: nutrition, exercises (which ones, how, and how many), time, planning, money, and motivation.

A great leader whom I work closely with always reminds me: "The confused mind says no. We reject what we can't or choose not to understand". Would you agree? I believe this is absolutely true. When we start to feel overwhelmed, we shrug off a real decision by answering, "I don't know."

My hope is that I am guiding you through a process that feels comfortable and doable for you. My methodology is just like my exercise regimens. If at any time you feel you need to increase the intensity, you are welcomed to spend more time in the journal.

If you feel something is too much for you to sort through, I encourage you to work on that assignment for a bit and return to it later that day for completion. I found that in creating this journal for you, my process is to share from my heart, pause, reflect, re-read and revisit. I encourage you to do the same. It is in doing so that we start to actualize our truths.

For this chapter's ending, I ask that you re-write your why and attach a S.M.A.R.T. Goal. What is a S.M.A.R.T goal? It is a goal that is Specific, Measurable, Attainable, Realistic and Time sensitive.

Do you have questions? Do you want to know why you have to re-do a task you have already done? You want to know what difference it makes if you have created a "dumb" goal or a "smart" goal? As long as you have a goal, right? Nope, wrong!

Two days ago, I warned you to grab a cup of tea and get ready because it was an important day. It was the day you developed and uncovered your "why". I hope it made you feel strongly about what is inspiring you as you thought it through. If it did not, I suggest you dig deeper into your initial why and readdress your answer.

You are now on Day 5. You have identified your why and your team. Now I want you to be more intentional. Remember, "someday" is not a goal. 50 pounds in 2 weeks is not realistic. "When hell freezes over" is not exactly an encouraging, time-sensitive deadline.

When you attach a S.M.A.R.T. goal to your why, it paints more of a complete picture. Once it is completed, you might say, "stuff just got real!".

For example, suppose your *why* is your realization that your weight is spiraling out of control. Say weight gain is starting to show not only on the scale but also via signs and symptoms of pre-diabetes, your goal may look like this:

"I will get healthy to reduce my risk of becoming diabetic".

Of course, this goal is a good start, but your goal needs to be *smarter*. If you have a goal without a deadline, it is simply a hope and if you have hope without a plan, it is simply a dream.

Your S.M.A.R.T. goal may look like this:

> *S. I will eat more natural fruits and vegetables and start exercising 3 days/week for 30 minutes*

> *M. I will start exercising 3 times a week for 30 mins*

> *A. I will release 7% of my body weight*

> *R. I will release 7% of my body weight or drop 2 sizes so I can feel good in my clothes*

> *T. In 3 months at my follow up appointment*

Can you see and hear the difference? The first goal is too generalized. I mean, who doesn't want to get healthy?

In all my years of caring for patients and training clients, I have never had one say to me, "I don't want to get healthy. I want to stay in this condition forever".

When you commit to adding specific values to your goals, you bring your *why* to life and it allows you to create a mini roadmap to your success.

DAY 5 - FIRST STEPS

1. Re-Write your WHY and attach a S.M.A.R.T Goal.

   S-specific/simple/significant
   M-measurable/meaningful
   A-attainable/achievable
   R-realistic/result oriented
   T-Time sensitive

Specific: _____

Measurable: _____

Achievable: _____

Realistic: _____

Time-Sensitive: _____

2. Exhale…You have completed day 5.

F.I.T. TIP:

If it doesn't challenge you, it won't change you.

DAY 6

"Persist in a state of perpetual preparation". I saw this quote on the Instagram account of one of my favorite bodybuilders, Kai Greene.

It is time to prepare your mind. Get your house in order. It's time to do the following:

- Create grocery lists
- Review healthy food options
- Practice label reading
- Purge the pantry
- Download *Beyond Diet* app or *My Fitness Pal* app (optional helpful tools)
- Purchase a food scale, bathroom scale, and measuring tape
- Join *Kimmy's Fitness Community (KFC)* on Facebook
- Opt in for my encouraging and helpful emails and videos at www.kimmyfitfitness.com

DAY 6 - FIRST STEPS

LABEL READING

Nutrition Facts

8 servings per container

Serving size   2/3 cup (55g)

Amount per serving

Calories   **230**

	% Daily Value*
Total Fat 8g	**10%**
Saturated Fat 1g	**5%**
Trans Fat 0g	
Cholesterol 0mg	**0%**
Sodium 160mg	**7%**
Total Carbohydrate 37g	**13%**
Dietary Fiber 4g	**14%**
Total Sugars 12g	
Includes 10g Added Sugars	**20%**
Protein 3g	
Vitamin D 2mcg	10%
Calcium 260mg	20%
Iron 8mg	45%
Potassium 235mg	6%

* The % Daily Value (DV) tells you how much a nutrient in a serving of food contributes to a daily diet. 2,000 calories a day is used for general nutrition advice.

A few things to consider as you head to the grocery store and attempt to make healthier choices. If you are new at understanding labels, the following are a few things to remember:

1.	**Servings per container** The number of servings in the entire container.
2.	**Serving size** How much is considered in one serving. Example: On this label, there are 8 total servings. 2/3 cup is one serving. That means there are 7 more servings left for consumption. There are 230 calories in one serving (2/3 cup). If you eat the entire container you will have consumed 1,840 calories (230 calories multiplied by 8 servings)! You will also be consuming 8 times the other listed nutrients - fat, cholesterol, sodium, carbohydrates, fiber, sugars, etc.
3.	**Calories** Listed PER serving. If you are trying to release weight, consider reducing your calorie intake by selecting foods with fewer calories per serving and be mindful of how much of the container you consume
4.	**Nutrients** One serving of food with 5% or less of the daily value is considered low. One serving of a food with 20% or more of the daily value is considered high. Be cognizant of limiting fat, cholesterol (less than 200mg / day if you have heart disease), carbohydrates and sugars. Aim to get more vitamins and minerals as they are very important nutrients

Document your Body Measurements

Weight   _____

Chest (across breast line)   _____

Neutral waist (at navel)   _____

Upper waistline   _____

Hips   _____

Each thigh (mid-thigh)   _____

Take these measurements once a week and DO NOT be consumed by numbers alone! Take all data inputs first thing in the morning upon awakening, after using the bathroom and before eating or drinking anything.

F.I.T. TIP:

The best project you'll ever work on is yourself.

DAY 7

F.I.T. COMMITMENT

I am starting this fitness journey on

_____

(Date)

I will join the *KFC* community for support any time I want because I do not have to do this alone. I will introduce myself and share with *KFC* why I opted to join the group so they can help me.

I am committed to completing the initial 30-day phase of this process because

_____

_____

_____

_____

_____

I am willing to trust the process and share my experiences as I am comfortable doing so (the good, bad and ugly) because

_____

_____

_____

_____

_____

I will not overeat. I will not under eat, over exercise or obsess over the scale. I will not live off excuses for 30 days because

_____

_____

_____

_____

I will not quit. I will encourage others not to quit. I will reach out to my support team when I feel stuck or discouraged because I know

_____

_____

_____

_____

I will frequently remind myself:

"When I limit what I WILL do, I limit the discovery of what I CAN do."

These are my commitments. I can and I will because health is what I AM.

Love,

_____

(sign your name)

Date _____

Supported by: Kimmy Ross

Your final commitment for Week 1 is the above *F.I.T. Commitment*. Complete it, rip it out and take it with you, post it or refer to it often. It is our paper "pinky promise".

You have completed the Free Health Assessment, your first week of journaling, and your F.I.T Commitment.

CONGRATULATIONS!

F.I.T. TIP:

When you open your eyes in the mornings, literally open your mouth and say something good about yourself, your life, your journey. I find this to be more powerful than just thinking it. Hearing your words, in your voice, makes you pay attention.

Warning! This could result in a full-blown empowering conversation with yourself!

CHAPTER 3:

PLANNING - Make It F.I.T.
(Finding Increments of Time)

Use the chart below, as well as the other charts within this journal to pencil in your weekly schedule. Feel free to make copies of the blank charts or create your own so that you can re-use them as you see fit.

Again, putting pen or pencil to paper is powerful. This will allow you to see every window of opportunity you have to make it F.I.T. We all have 1440 minutes in a day. How we choose to use that time is up to us.

Make It F.I.T. Schedule

	Sunday	Monday	Tuesday	Wednesday	Thursday	Friday	Saturday
6:00							
6:30							
7:00							
7:30							
8:00							
8:30							
9:00							
9:30							
10:00							

10:30							
11:00							
11:30							
12:00							
12:30							
1:00							
1:30							
2:00							
2:30							
3:00							
3:30							
4:00							
4:30							
5:00							
5:30							
6:00							
6:30							
7:00							
7:30							
8:00							
8:30							
9:00							
9:30							
10:00							

FOOD PREP

Most people who are new to the idea of the ever so popular "meal prepping" are unsure how or where to begin. I promise you that it is much like anything else. Once you learn some basic approaches to meal prepping, you will be able to adopt the habits easily and incorporate them in a way that works best for you and your family.

MEAL PREPARATION GUIDE

Invest in some good food containers, mostly the same size. I like the clear, preferably BPA-free ones with a good lid. They are reliable, I can see what's inside, and they will endure the microwave.

Also, Ziploc bags are the JAM! They come in many convenient sizes, even snack sizes. Buy a few boxes of these.

Grab your items from last week Day 6 (grocery list, label reading, healthy food options and food prep supply list) and let's get cooking! *Request your healthy food options via www.kimmyfitfitness.com

Using the healthy food list provided, decide on what you will be picking up from the market. Put some thought into what you will choose to eat during the week - breakfast, snack, lunch, snack, and dinner. This will make it easier to of it all once you unload the car and dive into your kitchen.

Many people choose Sunday and Wednesday as food preparation days. I suggest you do whatever is conducive to your lifestyle. When you prep on a Sunday, you can prepare enough food to last you until Wednesday and then on Wednesday you can prepare enough food for the remainder of the week.

You will be cooking food for macronutrients which are: protein, fats, and carbohydrates. Those will be your primary bulk items. You may already have favorite recipes or ingredients that you know you and your family will enjoy. I wouldn't remove those as options; however, if they are not healthier versions of your favorite dishes, research and consider how to swap a few ingredients for healthier alternatives.

This way you can still enjoy your favorite homemade sauces and marinades to be included in your meal preparation. No one is excited about eating the same exact thing every day, so be open to the possibilities of new culinary experiences.

Micronutrients are an important part of nutrition as well. Typically found in everyday foods or high-quality supplements, "micros" consist of vitamins and minerals such as iron, calcium, chromium, and zinc.

Micronutrients are essential elements to proper bodily functions like water balance, metabolism, cardiac rhythm, production of red blood cells, energy, growth, and development. Make sure you are consuming enough healthy and balanced calories.

F.I.T. MEALS

F.I.T. FITNESS	Breakfast	Snack	Lunch	Snack	Dinner	Snack (optional)
Sunday						
Monday						
Tuesday						
Wednesday						

Thursday						
Friday						
Saturday						
Don't forget to meal prep						

FOOD FOR THOUGHT

When you consider how foods are planted, produced and processed nowadays, many of the essential nutrients are lacking. I liken it to purchasing a new car. As you drive that car off the lot, it immediately loses its value. Same is true of most of our foods. Oranges shipped from Brazil lose their value from the time they are picked, packed, shipped, handled and delivered to your local grocer. It does not stop there.

Produce sit in boxes, on shelves, are exchanged hand to hand, dropped and restocked until they are finally purchased for consumption. Once you finally have those "fresh" oranges in your home, you decide if you will peel, juice, or simmer them in a savory citrus sauce. All of this impacts the nutritional integrity of the foods we eat.

What I am attempting to explain is, contrary to what some physicians may tell us, we are *not* getting all the nutrients we need from our food. Food alone is not enough.

I encourage you to check out the documentary called *Food Matters*, 2009, Written by Laurentine Ten Bosch. Directed by James Colquhoun and Carlo Ledesma. This will further substantiate the information revealed to you from the health assessment that you should have already taken, found at http://www.whynottry.idlife.com.

FOOD PREP HACKS

- Crockpots ROCK! Use them for healthy soups and complete meals.

- If cooking is not your strength, keep it simple. Start with recipes that require only a few ingredients or steps. Easy meal example: Chicken, potatoes, and green beans. Viola!

- Another quick hack is to pre-cut and clean all your chicken breasts and place them in small zip lock bags. Freeze the uncooked and unseasoned chicken until ready for use.

- Put chili powder or cayenne pepper on everything. It's a natural appetite suppressant and speeds up metabolism.

Be encouraged. Remember that some meal prep is better than none. There is no right or wrong way. You will figure out successful ways of working, if you start the work!

PROTEIN

- If you have chosen chicken breast as your lean protein for the week or part of the week, you can season, grill or bake all the chicken at one time. If you prefer a bit of variety in seasoning, you can opt to separate the chicken on the baking dish, distinguishing for yourself which pieces are seasoned with what.

Personally, I find it easy to line the chicken up in rows and stick to no more than a couple of flavors at one time.

- Seafood is another great lean protein option. I commonly choose whiting, flounder or salmon. I like to have my seafood made relatively fresh so if I cook this ahead of time, I aim to eat it within a day or so of preparation. Even if you have to cook it on the spot, seafood is a no-brainer and at least you will have your side dishes already prepared ahead of time.

CARBOHYDRATES

Let's address the big ole elephant in the room - Carbs (specifically starches). The most feared food group on the planet. Listen closely, carbs are our friend. You do not need to avoid them like the plague.

There are two types of carbohydrates - simple and complex carbohydrates. I believe the reason most people fear carbs or even blame carbs for all that goes wrong with their bodies is because of the lack of understanding of how to choose appropriate the carbs that can work in their favor.

All carbs are converted into simple sugars; however, simple carbs tend to cause higher spikes insulin production. When your insulin levels spike due to a rapid influx of sugar into the body, that sugar is most likely going to be deposited into fat cells. This is where you may notice yourself gaining weight/fat.

I do not encourage doing away with all carbs. There is plenty of research out there supporting the importance of carbs for people of different activity levels. Carbohydrates aid in the uptake of glycogen and serves as a source of energy. Carbs also act as a protein-sparing partner when consumed with protein. I would suggest including a complex carb with a low-fat protein option with most meals. These two nutritional sources complement each other. When you have enough carbs in your system, your body will pull it's energy from the carb source versus the protein source in your body. That's a good thing! You will be putting in a lot of hard work and you do not want to deplete the amino acids (the building blocks of protein) inside your muscles and cause any muscle depletion. There are other adverse side effects that can occur as a result of drastic carbohydrate depletion so I caution against doing so.

I will offer a caveat to this. If you are an advanced athlete in training, you will likely be advised by a coach or fitness professional in your sport to make adjustments to carbs, proteins, fats, as well as your overall caloric intake. For the purposes of this section of the F.I.T. journal, I am primarily addressing the "everyday" person seeking simple explanations of effective nutritional planning. Carbs are our friend!

Complex carbohydrates are easy to prepare. A large pot of brown rice, parboiled rice, quinoa. A large batch of roasted or oven baked sweet potatoes go a long way. YUM!!

VEGETABLES

Vegetables are always fun. I know what you are thinking: *This woman is so far gone in the fitness world that she has forgotten the real definition of fun*. No, I haven't. Veggies are FUN because you can get really creative with them, exploring new ways to season them with each meal. You also get to enjoy them freely without the risk of overly indulging in unwanted calories. This is where I break out my wok, apron, and fake Julia Child accent (yes, I feel quite fancy when I do).

TEMPERATURE CHECK

Be honest. How are you feeling about this? Let me give you some space to write it out…

1. What trepidations do you have concerning preparing your meals during the week?

_____

_____

_____

_____

2. What can you do that would be a reasonable start for you?

_____

_____

_____

_____

I want to reassure you that you do NOT have to prep your entire pantry. If the thought of preparing all your meals for 3-4 days at a time kills your vibe, then consider which meal(s) or mealtimes would make the most positive impact throughout your week. Do you struggle with specific meals, perhaps breakfast, snacking or dinnertime? Try tackling one or two of these problem areas during your first couple of weeks. Start simple.

WATER

Are you aware that 75% of most Americans are DEHYDRATED? It's true. It may be difficult to conceptualize, because people who are drinking sodas, flavored waters, sports drinks, and alcoholic beverages may consider those beverages as part of their daily hydration. Yes, some people think a cold beer is hydration. It is not.

We absolutely must talk about the importance of water intake. The truth of the matter is that sports drinks and similar products are doing more harm than good. These beverages are composed of large amounts of sugars, sugar substances and artificial additives. Keep in mind sometimes these sugary drinks contain *multiple* servings!

As a matter of fact, if you have not purged your pantry or fridge just yet, go grab a bottle and read the label. You will undoubtedly see sugar labelled as Sucralose, high fructose corn syrup, and fructose. It may even be listed under another name, as some other form of sugar. Many medical and scientific studies have identified sugar and artificial sweeteners like aspartame as proven carcinogens (cancer-causing agents) and neurotoxins. Sugar is also a highly addictive chemical with no nutritional benefits. The addictive properties of sugar affect pathways in the brain similar to those with addictions to heroin and morphine.

When we think about the composition of the human body, fifty-five to sixty-five percent of our body is composed of water. Water composition is generally higher in men (60%) because women tend to have more fatty tissue and fatty tissue contains less water than the lean tissue in men.

When we fail to properly hydrate our bodies, we become dehydrated. That is pretty straight forward. However, it gets complicated when the body needs to rely on food as its primary source of water (remember many of us have less than commendable diets).

Our brains do not make the distinction between hunger and thirst. When many of us are dehydrated, we may reach for food when in fact we are thirsty and our body is in need of water. When we reach for food and snacks instead of water, this leads to unnecessary caloric intake, promoting ongoing dehydration. Your thirsty body then begins pulling water from all other areas of the body causing water retention, resulting in weight gain.

In case you need more reasons to raise your glass, here are a few more benefits of water:

- Flushes toxins from the body
- Promotes regularity
- Improves energy
- Promotes weight loss
- Decreases headaches
- Improves skin complexion

If you are one of those people who struggle with water intake, here are a few tricks that may help:

- Add/Infuse your water with fruit slices and/or mint leaves.
- Drink water every time you think about it.
- Create water drinking habits (drink at every red light, during commercials, between exercise sets, etc.).
- Break your goal into smaller goals. Instead of visualizing the gallon of water you want to complete, break it down into 4 or 5 refillable 28 oz. shaker cups.
- Drink 8 oz. upon rising in the morning, 8 oz. with your vitamins, 8 oz. before each meal, and 8 oz. before bedtime.

Stepping up your fitness game means you will need to step up your water game as well. Sixty-four ounces (1/2 gallon) each day is a reasonable goal unless instructed otherwise. Some people consume that amount easily and some will exceed it.

Water is our most vital source of energy. Other than frequent bathroom visits, you will appreciate the positive effects of water to combat fatigue, hunger, joint discomfort and many other symptoms of dehydration throughout the day. I suggest you set 64 ounces as a goal if you are not there yet. If you have already reached 64 ounces and you are working out more frequently, at higher intensities and sweating more, change your goal to more than one gallon.

F.I.T. TIP:

If you find yourself joining your friends for happy hour, drinking 8 oz. of water in between your adult beverages will help you to pace alcohol intake and rehydrate in between beverages.

FOOD PREP CHECK-IN

What was your most proud food prep steps(s) this week?

_____

_____

_____

What was your biggest struggle or setback?

_____

_____

_____

What will you improve to avoid that struggle for next week?

_____

_____

_____

What will you plan to implement next week?

_____

_____

_____

F.I.T. TIP:

You don't have to create fancy or complicated masterpieces - just real food from fresh ingredients.

CHAPTER 4

MOVE IT OR LOSE IT.
HOW BADLY DO YOU WANT IT?

Are you ready? It is time to try a little bit harder. Come on. You didn't come this far to only come this far.

Remember this formula:
Nutrition is 80% / Exercise is 20% = Results.

I hope by now we have established some beginning level of trust and we can continue to move forward together. I am confident that now is a good time for you to start moving your body more if you haven't already started to do so.

Before starting any fitness regimen, I suggest you get clearance from a professional healthcare provider as warranted. This is to ensure that specific exercise programs are well suited for you. If you are currently dealing with some health or physical challenges, this does NOT mean you cannot exercise. It means you will need to make necessary adaptations and progress carefully for your safety.

Prior to jumping right into exercise, regardless of how excited you are to do so, it is always wise to prepare your body for what's to come. We do this by, of course, good nutrition and recovery, but also with proper stretching before and after killing your routine.

Take a moment to *Google* dynamic stretches. Dynamic stretches such as arm and shoulder circles, side bends, hip circles, leg swings and lunges are examples of good motion prior to the actual exercise routine.

Dynamic stretching is crucial before exercising and static exercises are also important afterwards. You can find examples of both via a *Google* search. Let us proceed to the workout I have created for you KFC style. It is delicious!

I want to share one of my High-Intensity Interval Training (HIIT) routines with you. These are tried and tested full body, compound (use of multiple joints at one time) exercises that I have used with clients who were either "recovering couch potatoes" or already active individuals seeking to push past a threshold or change up their routine.

Full body exercise routines simply make sense. They use compound movements that create balance in your physique, burns calories efficiently, build overall strength and eventually muscle mass gains.

In doing this KFC Challenge, members of my KFC private group reported feeling revived (a release of emotional fat) and challenged (a release of physical weight). Members reported releasing up to 6 pounds within a couple of weeks by just incorporating the challenge a few times a week in conjunction with what they were already doing or as a replacement for what they were doing. The KFC challenge along with the hydration challenge proved effective and inspiring.

The following challenge is purposed to give you a variety of exercises that you can work through over 15-20 minutes. Whether you categorize yourself as a beginner (affectionally referred to by me as my "recovering couch potato"), intermediate or advanced, you can use the KFC Challenge as your new baseline or new goal.

BEGINNER

I recommend attempting each move for as many repetitions as possible on your first attempt. Write the number of repetitions down in the journal. This is your baseline - your starting point. Do the same for the remaining exercises for the rest of the week. Listen to your body and take breaks as you need to.

After establishing all your baseline data, you will use those numbers as your goal for the following week. You will replace the numbers listed in the challenge with your baseline numbers for now. So, if you accomplished 5 pushups, 5 pushups are what you will execute for that exercise for the rest of that week and the next week.

You will complete each weekday working for at least 15-20 minutes through the round, taking rest breaks as needed. Challenge yourself to progress to intermediate level once the beginner's guidelines become less challenging for you.

INTERMEDIATE

Participants are recommended to strive for at least half of the repetitions indicated in the challenge and complete each workout on that weekday for at least 15-20 minutes with 15-30 seconds of rest between rounds.

Rest more if needed. Challenge yourself to progress to the advanced level once the intermediate guidelines become less challenging.

ADVANCED

Participants will strive to complete the challenge as outlined with 15-20 second breaks between rounds and working within the 20 minute timeframe. As part of your progression, try to squeeze in an additional round or two once the advanced guidelines become less challenging.

I encourage everyone to write down their accomplishments, no matter if they are big or small. Also, record what challenged you the most. How many rounds did you accomplish in your allotted timeframe? Did you track your heart rate? How did you feel afterwards?

Incorporate this challenge for 6-8 weeks along with increasing your water intake as previously discussed.

F.I.T. TIP:

Health, wellness, and fitness are not exclusive of each other. When you make the connection in understanding that your health status is truly the foundation of all you are able do, the more in tune you will become with your goals and the closer you will be to actualizing them.

---

4 WEEK CHALLENGE

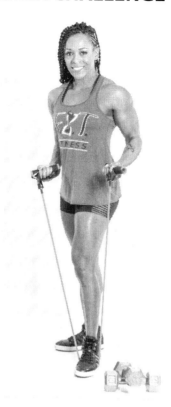

MONDAY	TUESDAY
10 push ups 20 body squats 30 crunches 30 bicycles 20 lunges 30 sec. high knees	30 sec. high knees 20 clapping jumping jacks 15 regular push ups 20 glute bridges 1-legged squats 10 each 10 jump squats 10 push ups

WEDNESDAY

15 Mountain Climbers
14 sumo squats
15 side crunches each side
30 sec. planks
20 jumping jacks
15 squats
25 V-up toe touches

THURSDAY

20 lunges
20 squats
10 push ups
10 1-leg glute bridge 10 each
20 Mtn. Climbers

FRIDAY

10 burpees
20 V-up toe touches
20 squats w/alternating side leg lift
10 push ups
10 burpees
30 bicycles

SATURDAY/SUNDAY

20-30 minutes
Cardio of choice

*WEEKEND CHECK-IN
*SATURDAY SELFIE

KIMMY'S KFC CHALLENGE

4 weeks KFC Progress:

F.I.T. FITNESS	Week 1	Week 2	Week 3	Week 4
# of COMPLETED ROUNDS				
TIME TO COMPLETION				
CHALLENGES				
SUCCESSES				

F.I.T. Tip
You got this. You can do anything, except quit.

CHAPTER 5
F.I.T. CHECK-INS (DAY 1-30)

DAY 1

FOOD PLAN
WHAT WILL I EAT TODAY?

Breakfast:
_____
_____

Snack:
_____
_____

Lunch:
_____
_____

Snack:
_____
_____

Dinner:
_____
_____

Snack (optional):
_____
_____

YOUR EXERCISE ACTION PLAN (Strength training, Cardio, Circuit, Yoga, etc.)

_____

_____

EXPLAIN YOUR FEELINGS AND THOUGHTS BEFORE EXERCISE (Happy, Excited, Tired, Frustrated)

_____

_____

_____

WHAT WERE YOUR CHALLENGES DURING EXERCISE?

_____

_____

EXPLAIN YOUR THOUGHTS AND FEELINGS AFTER EXERCISE (Confident, Disappointed, Excited, Energized)

_____

_____

WHAT DID YOU DO WELL?

_____

_____

WHAT DIDN'T QUITE F.I.T. OR NEEDS TO CHANGE?

_____

_____

DAY 2

FOOD PLAN
WHAT WILL I EAT TODAY?

Breakfast:
_____
_____
_____

Snack:
_____
_____
_____

Lunch:
_____
_____
_____

Snack:
_____
_____
_____

Dinner:
_____
_____
_____

Snack (optional):
_____
_____
_____

YOUR EXERCISE ACTION PLAN (Strength training, Cardio, Circuit, Yoga, etc.)

_____

_____

EXPLAIN YOUR FEELINGS AND THOUGHTS BEFORE EXERCISE (Happy, Excited, Tired, Frustrated)

_____

_____

_____

WHAT WERE YOUR CHALLENGES DURING EXERCISE?

_____

_____

EXPLAIN YOUR THOUGHTS AND FEELINGS AFTER EXERCISE (Confident, Disappointed, Excited, Energized)

_____

_____

WHAT DID YOU DO WELL?

_____

_____

WHAT DIDN'T QUITE F.I.T. OR NEEDS TO CHANGE?

_____

_____

DAY 3

FOOD PLAN
WHAT WILL I EAT TODAY?

Breakfast:

_____

_____

Snack:

_____

_____

Lunch:

_____

_____

Snack:

_____

_____

Dinner:

_____

_____

Snack (optional):

_____

_____

_____

YOUR EXERCISE ACTION PLAN (Strength training, Cardio, Circuit, Yoga, etc.)

_____

_____

EXPLAIN YOUR FEELINGS AND THOUGHTS BEFORE EXERCISE (Happy, Excited, Tired, Frustrated)

_____

_____

_____

WHAT WERE YOUR CHALLENGES DURING EXERCISE?

_____

_____

EXPLAIN YOUR THOUGHTS AND FEELINGS AFTER EXERCISE (Confident, Disappointed, Excited, Energized)

_____

_____

WHAT DID YOU DO WELL?

_____

_____

WHAT DIDN'T QUITE F.I.T. OR NEEDS TO CHANGE?

_____

_____

NOT F.I.T. FOR EMOTIONAL FAT:

Love yourself enough so that you require less approval from others.

DAY 4

FOOD PLAN
WHAT WILL I EAT TODAY?

Breakfast:
_____
_____
_____

Snack:
_____
_____
_____

Lunch:
_____
_____
_____

Snack:
_____
_____
_____

Dinner:
_____
_____
_____

Snack (optional):
_____
_____
_____

YOUR EXERCISE ACTION PLAN (Strength training, Cardio, Circuit, Yoga, etc.)

_____

_____

EXPLAIN YOUR FEELINGS AND THOUGHTS BEFORE EXERCISE (Happy, Excited, Tired, Frustrated)

_____

_____

_____

WHAT WERE YOUR CHALLENGES DURING EXERCISE?

_____

_____

EXPLAIN YOUR THOUGHTS AND FEELINGS AFTER EXERCISE (Confident, Disappointed, Excited, Energized)

_____

_____

WHAT DID YOU DO WELL?

_____

_____

WHAT DIDN'T QUITE F.I.T. OR NEEDS TO CHANGE?

_____

_____

DAY 5

FOOD PLAN
WHAT WILL I EAT TODAY?

Breakfast:

_____

_____

Snack:

_____

_____

Lunch:

_____

_____

Snack:

_____

_____

Dinner:

_____

_____

Snack (optional):

_____

_____

YOUR EXERCISE ACTION PLAN (Strength training, Cardio, Circuit, Yoga, etc.)

_____

_____

EXPLAIN YOUR FEELINGS AND THOUGHTS BEFORE EXERCISE (Happy, Excited, Tired, Frustrated)

_____

_____

_____

WHAT WERE YOUR CHALLENGES DURING EXERCISE?

_____

_____

EXPLAIN YOUR THOUGHTS AND FEELINGS AFTER EXERCISE (Confident, Disappointed, Excited, Energized)

_____

_____

WHAT DID YOU DO WELL?

_____

_____

WHAT DIDN'T QUITE F.I.T. OR NEEDS TO CHANGE?

_____

_____

DAY 6

FOOD PLAN
WHAT WILL I EAT TODAY?

Breakfast:
_____
_____

Snack:
_____
_____

Lunch:
_____
_____

Snack:
_____
_____

Dinner:
_____
_____

Snack (optional):
_____
_____

YOUR EXERCISE ACTION PLAN (Strength training, Cardio, Circuit, Yoga, etc.)

_____

_____

EXPLAIN YOUR FEELINGS AND THOUGHTS BEFORE EXERCISE (Happy, Excited, Tired, Frustrated)

_____

_____

_____

WHAT WERE YOUR CHALLENGES DURING EXERCISE?

_____

_____

EXPLAIN YOUR THOUGHTS AND FEELINGS AFTER EXERCISE (Confident, Disappointed, Excited, Energized)

_____

_____

WHAT DID YOU DO WELL?

_____

_____

WHAT DIDN'T QUITE F.I.T. OR NEEDS TO CHANGE?

_____

_____

NOT F.I.T. FOR EMOTIONAL FAT:

Stop trying to prove that you are good and good enough.
Just know that you are.

DAY 7

FOOD PLAN
WHAT WILL I EAT TODAY?

Breakfast:
_____
_____
_____

Snack:
_____
_____
_____

Lunch:
_____
_____
_____

Snack:
_____
_____
_____

Dinner:
_____
_____
_____

Snack (optional):
_____
_____
_____

YOUR EXERCISE ACTION PLAN (Strength training, Cardio, Circuit, Yoga, etc.)

_____

_____

EXPLAIN YOUR FEELINGS AND THOUGHTS BEFORE EXERCISE (Happy, Excited, Tired, Frustrated)

_____

_____

_____

WHAT WERE YOUR CHALLENGES DURING EXERCISE?

_____

_____

EXPLAIN YOUR THOUGHTS AND FEELINGS AFTER EXERCISE (Confident, Disappointed, Excited, Energized)

_____

_____

WHAT DID YOU DO WELL?

_____

_____

WHAT DIDN'T QUITE F.I.T. OR NEEDS TO CHANGE?

_____

_____

DAY 8

FOOD PLAN
WHAT WILL I EAT TODAY?

Breakfast:

_____

_____

_____

Snack:

_____

_____

_____

Lunch:

_____

_____

_____

Snack:

_____

_____

_____

Dinner:

_____

_____

_____

Snack (optional):

_____

_____

_____

YOUR EXERCISE ACTION PLAN (Strength training, Cardio, Circuit, Yoga, etc.)

_____

_____

EXPLAIN YOUR FEELINGS AND THOUGHTS BEFORE EXERCISE (Happy, Excited, Tired, Frustrated)

_____

_____

_____

WHAT WERE YOUR CHALLENGES DURING EXERCISE?

_____

_____

EXPLAIN YOUR THOUGHTS AND FEELINGS AFTER EXERCISE (Confident, Disappointed, Excited, Energized)

_____

_____

WHAT DID YOU DO WELL?

_____

_____

WHAT DIDN'T QUITE F.I.T. OR NEEDS TO CHANGE?

_____

_____

DAY 9

Breakfast:

_____
_____
_____

Snack:

_____
_____
_____

Lunch:

_____
_____
_____

Snack:

_____
_____
_____

Dinner:

_____
_____
_____

Snack (optional):

_____
_____
_____

YOUR EXERCISE ACTION PLAN (Strength training, Cardio, Circuit, Yoga, etc.)

_____

_____

EXPLAIN YOUR FEELINGS AND THOUGHTS BEFORE EXERCISE (Happy, Excited, Tired, Frustrated)

_____

_____

_____

WHAT WERE YOUR CHALLENGES DURING EXERCISE?

_____

_____

EXPLAIN YOUR THOUGHTS AND FEELINGS AFTER EXERCISE (Confident, Disappointed, Excited, Energized)

_____

_____

WHAT DID YOU DO WELL?

_____

_____

WHAT DIDN'T QUITE F.I.T. OR NEEDS TO CHANGE?

_____

_____

NOT F.I.T. FOR EMOTIONAL FAT:

"That which you allow will eventually show up at your door." - Suzan Hart
Stand up for people and principles. Do this because you understand too well what it feels like to have no one stand up for you.

DAY 10

FOOD PLAN
WHAT WILL I EAT TODAY?

Breakfast:

_____
_____
_____

Snack:

_____
_____
_____

Lunch:

_____
_____
_____

Snack:

_____
_____
_____

Dinner:

_____
_____
_____

Snack (optional):

_____
_____
_____

YOUR EXERCISE ACTION PLAN (Strength training, Cardio, Circuit, Yoga, etc.)

_____

_____

EXPLAIN YOUR FEELINGS AND THOUGHTS BEFORE EXERCISE (Happy, Excited, Tired, Frustrated)

_____

_____

_____

WHAT WERE YOUR CHALLENGES DURING EXERCISE?

_____

_____

EXPLAIN YOUR THOUGHTS AND FEELINGS AFTER EXERCISE (Confident, Disappointed, Excited, Energized)

_____

_____

WHAT DID YOU DO WELL?

_____

_____

WHAT DIDN'T QUITE F.I.T. OR NEEDS TO CHANGE?

_____

_____

DAY 11

FOOD PLAN
WHAT WILL I EAT TODAY?

Breakfast:

_____
_____
_____

Snack:

_____
_____
_____

Lunch:

_____
_____
_____

Snack:

_____
_____
_____

Dinner:

_____
_____
_____

Snack (optional):

_____
_____
_____

YOUR EXERCISE ACTION PLAN (Strength training, Cardio, Circuit, Yoga, etc.)

_____

_____

EXPLAIN YOUR FEELINGS AND THOUGHTS BEFORE EXERCISE (Happy, Excited, Tired, Frustrated)

_____

_____

_____

WHAT WERE YOUR CHALLENGES DURING EXERCISE?

_____

_____

EXPLAIN YOUR THOUGHTS AND FEELINGS AFTER EXERCISE (Confident, Disappointed, Excited, Energized)

_____

_____

WHAT DID YOU DO WELL?

_____

_____

WHAT DIDN'T QUITE F.I.T. OR NEEDS TO CHANGE?

_____

_____

DAY 12

FOOD PLAN
WHAT WILL I EAT TODAY?

Breakfast:

_____
_____
_____

Snack:

_____
_____
_____

Lunch:

_____
_____
_____

Snack:

_____
_____
_____

Dinner:

_____
_____
_____

Snack (optional):

_____
_____
_____

YOUR EXERCISE ACTION PLAN (Strength training, Cardio, Circuit, Yoga, etc.)

_____

_____

EXPLAIN YOUR FEELINGS AND THOUGHTS BEFORE EXERCISE (Happy, Excited, Tired, Frustrated)

_____

_____

_____

WHAT WERE YOUR CHALLENGES DURING EXERCISE?

_____

_____

EXPLAIN YOUR THOUGHTS AND FEELINGS AFTER EXERCISE (Confident, Disappointed, Excited, Energized)

_____

_____

WHAT DID YOU DO WELL?

_____

_____

WHAT DIDN'T QUITE F.I.T. OR NEEDS TO CHANGE?

_____

_____

NOT F.I.T. FOR EMOTIONAL FAT:

"Use who God sends you." It may not be your family or friends, but you are blessed and blessings abound. Keep fighting through the emotional fat and allow yourself to see them.

DAY 13

FOOD PLAN
WHAT WILL I EAT TODAY?

Breakfast:

_____
_____
_____

Snack:

_____
_____
_____

Lunch:

_____
_____
_____

Snack:

_____
_____
_____

Dinner:

_____
_____
_____

Snack (optional):

_____
_____
_____

YOUR EXERCISE ACTION PLAN (Strength training, Cardio, Circuit, Yoga, etc.)

EXPLAIN YOUR FEELINGS AND THOUGHTS BEFORE EXERCISE (Happy, Excited, Tired, Frustrated)

WHAT WERE YOUR CHALLENGES DURING EXERCISE?

EXPLAIN YOUR THOUGHTS AND FEELINGS AFTER EXERCISE (Confident, Disappointed, Excited, Energized)

WHAT DID YOU DO WELL?

WHAT DIDN'T QUITE F.I.T. OR NEEDS TO CHANGE?

DAY 14

FOOD PLAN
WHAT WILL I EAT TODAY?

Breakfast:

_____
_____
_____

Snack:

_____
_____
_____

Lunch:

_____
_____
_____

Snack:

_____
_____
_____

Dinner:

_____
_____
_____

Snack (optional):

_____
_____
_____

YOUR EXERCISE ACTION PLAN (Strength training, Cardio, Circuit, Yoga, etc.)

_____

_____

EXPLAIN YOUR FEELINGS AND THOUGHTS BEFORE EXERCISE (Happy, Excited, Tired, Frustrated)

_____

_____

_____

WHAT WERE YOUR CHALLENGES DURING EXERCISE?

_____

_____

EXPLAIN YOUR THOUGHTS AND FEELINGS AFTER EXERCISE (Confident, Disappointed, Excited, Energized)

_____

_____

WHAT DID YOU DO WELL?

_____

_____

WHAT DIDN'T QUITE F.I.T. OR NEEDS TO CHANGE?

_____

_____

DAY 15

FOOD PLAN
WHAT WILL I EAT TODAY?

Breakfast:

_____
_____
_____

Snack:

_____
_____
_____

Lunch:

_____
_____
_____

Snack:

_____
_____
_____

Dinner:

_____
_____
_____

Snack (optional):

_____
_____
_____

YOUR EXERCISE ACTION PLAN (Strength training, Cardio, Circuit, Yoga, etc.)

_____

_____

EXPLAIN YOUR FEELINGS AND THOUGHTS BEFORE EXERCISE (Happy, Excited, Tired, Frustrated)

_____

_____

_____

WHAT WERE YOUR CHALLENGES DURING EXERCISE?

_____

_____

EXPLAIN YOUR THOUGHTS AND FEELINGS AFTER EXERCISE (Confident, Disappointed, Excited, Energized)

_____

_____

WHAT DID YOU DO WELL?

_____

_____

WHAT DIDN'T QUITE F.I.T. OR NEEDS TO CHANGE?

_____

_____

NOT F.I.T. FOR EMOTIONAL FAT:

These are your goals and you have everything you need to accomplish them. Everyone will not understand, but I am cheering for YOU.

DAY 16

FOOD PLAN
WHAT WILL I EAT TODAY?

Breakfast:

_____

_____

_____

Snack:

_____

_____

_____

Lunch:

_____

_____

_____

Snack:

_____

_____

_____

Dinner:

_____

_____

_____

Snack (optional):

_____

_____

_____

YOUR EXERCISE ACTION PLAN (Strength training, Cardio, Circuit, Yoga, etc.)

_____

_____

EXPLAIN YOUR FEELINGS AND THOUGHTS BEFORE EXERCISE (Happy, Excited, Tired, Frustrated)

_____

_____

_____

WHAT WERE YOUR CHALLENGES DURING EXERCISE?

_____

_____

EXPLAIN YOUR THOUGHTS AND FEELINGS AFTER EXERCISE (Confident, Disappointed, Excited, Energized)

_____

_____

WHAT DID YOU DO WELL?

_____

_____

WHAT DIDN'T QUITE F.I.T. OR NEEDS TO CHANGE?

_____

_____

DAY 17

FOOD PLAN
WHAT WILL I EAT TODAY?

Breakfast:

_____
_____
_____

Snack:

_____
_____
_____

Lunch:

_____
_____
_____

Snack:

_____
_____
_____

Dinner:

_____
_____
_____

Snack (optional):

_____
_____
_____

YOUR EXERCISE ACTION PLAN (Strength training, Cardio, Circuit, Yoga, etc.)

_____

_____

EXPLAIN YOUR FEELINGS AND THOUGHTS BEFORE EXERCISE (Happy, Excited, Tired, Frustrated)

_____

_____

_____

WHAT WERE YOUR CHALLENGES DURING EXERCISE?

_____

_____

EXPLAIN YOUR THOUGHTS AND FEELINGS AFTER EXERCISE (Confident, Disappointed, Excited, Energized)

_____

_____

WHAT DID YOU DO WELL?

_____

_____

WHAT DIDN'T QUITE F.I.T. OR NEEDS TO CHANGE?

_____

_____

DAY 18

FOOD PLAN
WHAT WILL I EAT TODAY?

Breakfast:

_____

_____

_____

Snack:

_____

_____

_____

Lunch:

_____

_____

_____

Snack:

_____

_____

_____

Dinner:

_____

_____

_____

Snack (optional):

_____

_____

_____

YOUR EXERCISE ACTION PLAN (Strength training, Cardio, Circuit, Yoga, etc.)

_____

_____

EXPLAIN YOUR FEELINGS AND THOUGHTS BEFORE EXERCISE (Happy, Excited, Tired, Frustrated)

_____

_____

_____

WHAT WERE YOUR CHALLENGES DURING EXERCISE?

_____

_____

EXPLAIN YOUR THOUGHTS AND FEELINGS AFTER EXERCISE (Confident, Disappointed, Excited, Energized)

_____

_____

WHAT DID YOU DO WELL?

_____

_____

WHAT DIDN'T QUITE F.I.T. OR NEEDS TO CHANGE?

_____

_____

NOT F.I.T. FOR EMOTIONAL FAT:

It is too painstaking to try to be where you are not wanted or accepted. Follow the love instead.

DAY 19

FOOD PLAN
WHAT WILL I EAT TODAY?

Breakfast:

_____

_____

Snack:

_____

_____

Lunch:

_____

_____

Snack:

_____

_____

Dinner:

_____

_____

Snack (optional):

_____

_____

_____

YOUR EXERCISE ACTION PLAN (Strength training, Cardio, Circuit, Yoga, etc.)

_____

_____

EXPLAIN YOUR FEELINGS AND THOUGHTS BEFORE EXERCISE (Happy, Excited, Tired, Frustrated)

_____

_____

_____

WHAT WERE YOUR CHALLENGES DURING EXERCISE?

_____

_____

EXPLAIN YOUR THOUGHTS AND FEELINGS AFTER EXERCISE (Confident, Disappointed, Excited, Energized)

_____

_____

WHAT DID YOU DO WELL?

_____

_____

WHAT DIDN'T QUITE F.I.T. OR NEEDS TO CHANGE?

_____

_____

DAY 20

FOOD PLAN
WHAT WILL I EAT TODAY?

Breakfast:
_____
_____
_____

Snack:
_____
_____
_____

Lunch:
_____
_____
_____

Snack:
_____
_____
_____

Dinner:
_____
_____
_____

Snack (optional):
_____
_____
_____

YOUR EXERCISE ACTION PLAN (Strength training, Cardio, Circuit, Yoga, etc.)

_____

_____

EXPLAIN YOUR FEELINGS AND THOUGHTS BEFORE EXERCISE (Happy, Excited, Tired, Frustrated)

_____

_____

_____

WHAT WERE YOUR CHALLENGES DURING EXERCISE?

_____

_____

EXPLAIN YOUR THOUGHTS AND FEELINGS AFTER EXERCISE (Confident, Disappointed, Excited, Energized)

_____

_____

WHAT DID YOU DO WELL?

_____

_____

WHAT DIDN'T QUITE F.I.T. OR NEEDS TO CHANGE?

_____

_____

DAY 21

FOOD PLAN
WHAT WILL I EAT TODAY?

Breakfast:
_____
_____
_____

Snack:
_____
_____
_____

Lunch:
_____
_____
_____

Snack:
_____
_____
_____

Dinner:
_____
_____
_____

Snack (optional):
_____
_____
_____

YOUR EXERCISE ACTION PLAN (Strength training, Cardio, Circuit, Yoga, etc.)

_____

_____

EXPLAIN YOUR FEELINGS AND THOUGHTS BEFORE EXERCISE (Happy, Excited, Tired, Frustrated)

_____

_____

_____

WHAT WERE YOUR CHALLENGES DURING EXERCISE?

_____

_____

EXPLAIN YOUR THOUGHTS AND FEELINGS AFTER EXERCISE (Confident, Disappointed, Excited, Energized)

_____

_____

WHAT DID YOU DO WELL?

_____

_____

WHAT DIDN'T QUITE F.I.T. OR NEEDS TO CHANGE?

_____

_____

NOT F.I.T. FOR EMOTIONAL FAT:

It does not matter if your parents did not plan for your birth. God planned you and has plans for you. You better live!

...DAY 21 (3 WEEKS)

Oh My Gosh! Are you excited? Do you see how far along you have come?

STRIKE A POSE! DO IT! YOU DESERVE IT!

Okay, let's finish this last week strong. You are developing consistent habits and working through some of that emotional and physical fat. It's all helping you to visualize and become your healthier self.

Perhaps at this point you are stuck and unsure of what else you could be or should be doing, or maybe you are doing great and want to keep moving forward. I am good with wherever you have found yourself, as long as you are still turning the page each day (literally and figuratively). Hopefully by now, you are seeing that you have set some fitness goals along the way. What you are creating is a healthier lifestyle. Can you see the difference?

I am adding some exercise options for you to consider incorporating into your new lifestyle. Google and YouTube will be your friend for all of these:

- Dynamic stretches - We covered earlier
- Shoulders - Shoulder dumbbell presses, dumbbell shoulder raises to the side and to the front
- Arms (Biceps/Triceps Muscles) - Bicep curls with dumbbells or a weighted bar, triceps extensions, triceps kickbacks, triceps dips
- Chest - Dumbbell chest presses on the floor, dumbbell fly with dumbbells, pushups on knees or toes
- Back - Dumbbell single or double-arm rows, dumbbell bent over rows

- Stomach (Abdominal/Core Muscles) - Reverse crunches, lying v-up toe touches, Russian twists, sit ups, planks
- Legs (Quadricep/Hamstring Muscles) - Body weight squats, one leg squats, lunges (forward and backwards), jump squats
- Booty (Gluteal Muscles) - Donkey kickbacks, fire hydrants, glute bridges
- Calves - Standing calf raises (one leg or both, with weights or without)
- Static stretches - We covered earlier

F.I.T. TIP:

1 GRAM OF PROTEIN = 6 CALORIES
1 GRAM OF FAT = 9 CALORIES
1 GRAM OF CARBOHYDRATES = 6 CALORIES

DAY 22

YOUR EXERCISE ACTION PLAN (Strength training, Cardio, Circuit, Yoga, etc.)

_____

_____

EXPLAIN YOUR FEELINGS AND THOUGHTS BEFORE EXERCISE (Happy, Excited, Tired, Frustrated)

_____

_____

WHAT WERE YOUR CHALLENGES DURING EXERCISE

_____

_____

EXPLAIN YOUR THOUGHTS AND FEELINGS AFTER EXERCISE (Confident, Disappointed, Excited, Energized)

_____

_____

WHAT DID YOU DO WELL?

_____

_____

WHAT DIDN'T QUITE F.I.T. OR NEEDS TO CHANGE?

_____

_____

FOOD PLAN
WHAT WILL I EAT TODAY?

Breakfast:

_____
_____
_____

Snack:

_____
_____
_____

Lunch:

_____
_____
_____

Snack:

_____
_____
_____

Dinner:

_____

FOOD PLAN
WHAT WILL I EAT TODAY?

Breakfast:

_____
_____
_____

Snack:

_____

Lunch:

Snack:

Dinner:

Snack (optional):

YOUR EXERCISE ACTION PLAN (Strength training, Cardio, Circuit, Yoga, etc.)

_____

_____

EXPLAIN YOUR FEELINGS AND THOUGHTS BEFORE EXERCISE (Happy, Excited, Tired, Frustrated)

_____

_____

_____

WHAT WERE YOUR CHALLENGES DURING EXERCISE?

_____

_____

EXPLAIN YOUR THOUGHTS AND FEELINGS AFTER EXERCISE (Confident, Disappointed, Excited, Energized)

_____

_____

WHAT DID YOU DO WELL?

_____

_____

WHAT DIDN'T QUITE F.I.T. OR NEEDS TO CHANGE?

_____

_____

DAY 23

FOOD PLAN
WHAT WILL I EAT TODAY?

Breakfast:

_____

_____

_____

Snack:

_____

_____

_____

Lunch:

_____

_____

_____

Snack:

_____

_____

_____

Dinner:

_____

_____

_____

Snack (optional):

_____

_____

_____

YOUR EXERCISE ACTION PLAN (Strength training, Cardio, Circuit, Yoga, etc.)

_____

_____

EXPLAIN YOUR FEELINGS AND THOUGHTS BEFORE EXERCISE (Happy, Excited, Tired, Frustrated)

_____

_____

_____

WHAT WERE YOUR CHALLENGES DURING EXERCISE?

_____

_____

EXPLAIN YOUR THOUGHTS AND FEELINGS AFTER EXERCISE (Confident, Disappointed, Excited, Energized)

_____

_____

WHAT DID YOU DO WELL?

_____

_____

WHAT DIDN'T QUITE F.I.T. OR NEEDS TO CHANGE?

_____

_____

DAY 24

FOOD PLAN
WHAT WILL I EAT TODAY?

Breakfast:

_____
_____
_____

Snack:

_____
_____
_____

Lunch:

_____
_____
_____

Snack:

_____
_____
_____

Dinner:

_____
_____
_____

Snack (optional):

_____
_____
_____

YOUR EXERCISE ACTION PLAN (Strength training, Cardio, Circuit, Yoga, etc.)

_____

_____

EXPLAIN YOUR FEELINGS AND THOUGHTS BEFORE EXERCISE (Happy, Excited, Tired, Frustrated)

_____

_____

_____

WHAT WERE YOUR CHALLENGES DURING EXERCISE?

_____

_____

EXPLAIN YOUR THOUGHTS AND FEELINGS AFTER EXERCISE (Confident, Disappointed, Excited, Energized)

_____

_____

WHAT DID YOU DO WELL?

_____

_____

WHAT DIDN'T QUITE F.I.T. OR NEEDS TO CHANGE?

_____

_____

NOT F.I.T. FOR EMOTIONAL FAT:

Stop trying to prove that you are good and good enough.
Just know that you are.

DAY 25

FOOD PLAN
WHAT WILL I EAT TODAY?

Breakfast:

_____

_____

_____

Snack:

_____

_____

_____

Lunch:

_____

_____

_____

Snack:

_____

_____

_____

Dinner:

_____

_____

_____

Snack (optional):

_____

_____

_____

YOUR EXERCISE ACTION PLAN (Strength training, Cardio, Circuit, Yoga, etc.)

_____

_____

EXPLAIN YOUR FEELINGS AND THOUGHTS BEFORE EXERCISE (Happy, Excited, Tired, Frustrated)

_____

_____

_____

WHAT WERE YOUR CHALLENGES DURING EXERCISE?

_____

_____

EXPLAIN YOUR THOUGHTS AND FEELINGS AFTER EXERCISE (Confident, Disappointed, Excited, Energized)

_____

_____

WHAT DID YOU DO WELL?

_____

_____

WHAT DIDN'T QUITE F.I.T. OR NEEDS TO CHANGE?

_____

_____

DAY 26

FOOD PLAN
WHAT WILL I EAT TODAY?

Breakfast:

_____
_____
_____

Snack:

_____
_____
_____

Lunch:

_____
_____
_____

Snack:

_____
_____
_____

Dinner:

_____
_____
_____

Snack (optional):

_____
_____
_____

YOUR EXERCISE ACTION PLAN (Strength training, Cardio, Circuit, Yoga, etc.)

_____

_____

EXPLAIN YOUR FEELINGS AND THOUGHTS BEFORE EXERCISE (Happy, Excited, Tired, Frustrated)

_____

_____

_____

WHAT WERE YOUR CHALLENGES DURING EXERCISE?

_____

_____

EXPLAIN YOUR THOUGHTS AND FEELINGS AFTER EXERCISE (Confident, Disappointed, Excited, Energized)

_____

_____

WHAT DID YOU DO WELL?

_____

_____

WHAT DIDN'T QUITE F.I.T. OR NEEDS TO CHANGE?

_____

_____

DAY 27

FOOD PLAN
WHAT WILL I EAT TODAY?

Breakfast:

_____

_____

_____

Snack:

_____

_____

_____

Lunch:

_____

_____

_____

Snack:

_____

_____

_____

Dinner:

_____

_____

_____

Snack (optional):

_____

_____

_____

YOUR EXERCISE ACTION PLAN (Strength training, Cardio, Circuit, Yoga, etc.)

_____

_____

EXPLAIN YOUR FEELINGS AND THOUGHTS BEFORE EXERCISE (Happy, Excited, Tired, Frustrated)

_____

_____

_____

WHAT WERE YOUR CHALLENGES DURING EXERCISE?

_____

_____

EXPLAIN YOUR THOUGHTS AND FEELINGS AFTER EXERCISE (Confident, Disappointed, Excited, Energized)

_____

_____

WHAT DID YOU DO WELL?

_____

_____

WHAT DIDN'T QUITE F.I.T. OR NEEDS TO CHANGE?

_____

_____

NOT F.I.T. FOR EMOTIONAL FAT:

It's not okay to make excuses for yourself, but it is okay to forgive yourself.

DAY 28

FOOD PLAN
WHAT WILL I EAT TODAY?

Breakfast:

_____

_____

Snack:

_____

_____

Lunch:

_____

_____

Snack:

_____

_____

Dinner:

_____

_____

Snack (optional):

_____

_____

_____

YOUR EXERCISE ACTION PLAN (Strength training, Cardio, Circuit, Yoga, etc.)

_____

_____

EXPLAIN YOUR FEELINGS AND THOUGHTS BEFORE EXERCISE (Happy, Excited, Tired, Frustrated)

_____

_____

_____

WHAT WERE YOUR CHALLENGES DURING EXERCISE?

_____

_____

EXPLAIN YOUR THOUGHTS AND FEELINGS AFTER EXERCISE (Confident, Disappointed, Excited, Energized)

_____

_____

WHAT DID YOU DO WELL?

_____

_____

WHAT DIDN'T QUITE F.I.T. OR NEEDS TO CHANGE?

_____

_____

DAY 29

FOOD PLAN
WHAT WILL I EAT TODAY?

Breakfast:

_____

_____

_____

Snack:

_____

_____

_____

Lunch:

_____

_____

_____

Snack:

_____

_____

_____

Dinner:

_____

_____

_____

Snack (optional):

_____

_____

_____

YOUR EXERCISE ACTION PLAN (Strength training, Cardio, Circuit, Yoga, etc.)

_____

_____

EXPLAIN YOUR FEELINGS AND THOUGHTS BEFORE EXERCISE (Happy, Excited, Tired, Frustrated)

_____

_____

_____

WHAT WERE YOUR CHALLENGES DURING EXERCISE?

_____

_____

EXPLAIN YOUR THOUGHTS AND FEELINGS AFTER EXERCISE (Confident, Disappointed, Excited, Energized)

_____

_____

WHAT DID YOU DO WELL?

_____

_____

WHAT DIDN'T QUITE F.I.T. OR NEEDS TO CHANGE?

_____

_____

DAY 30

FOOD PLAN
WHAT WILL I EAT TODAY?

Breakfast:

_____

_____

_____

Snack:

_____

_____

_____

Lunch:

_____

_____

_____

Snack:

_____

_____

_____

Dinner:

_____

_____

_____

Snack (optional):

_____

_____

_____

YOUR EXERCISE ACTION PLAN (Strength training, Cardio, Circuit, Yoga, etc.)

_____

_____

EXPLAIN YOUR FEELINGS AND THOUGHTS BEFORE EXERCISE (Happy, Excited, Tired, Frustrated)

_____

_____

_____

WHAT WERE YOUR CHALLENGES DURING EXERCISE?

_____

_____

EXPLAIN YOUR THOUGHTS AND FEELINGS AFTER EXERCISE (Confident, Disappointed, Excited, Energized)

_____

_____

WHAT DID YOU DO WELL?

_____

_____

WHAT DIDN'T QUITE F.I.T. OR NEEDS TO CHANGE?

_____

_____

NOT F.I.T. FOR EMOTIONAL FAT:

The opinions of others will change in an instant. Do not let their compliments take you too high and do not let their criticisms take you under.

CONGRATULATIONS!!!
JOURNEY TO BE CONTINUED...

My heart is full of happiness for you. I hope you are as excited and inspired as I am about this journey we have taken together. I have thought about each of you who have purchased this journal.

I want to thank **YOU** personally. If it helped you in some way and you are confident that my *F.I.T. Journal* could also help someone you know, please shout from a mountain top about how this is a *must-have*.

Okay, maybe that's a big request. I just figured that since you've made it this far, a mountain top would be a piece of cake (pun intended). Seriously, thank you in advance for your endorsement and referrals. I am blessed to be a blessing. To quote another memorable figure, Marilyn Monroe, "*I just want to be great*" and I want the same for you.

Let me know how you are doing. Tweet me, follow me, sign up for my email list at **www.kimmyfitfitness.com**.

You can learn more about healthy nutrition and fitness options customized for you, as well as natural performance and weight loss products at my nutrition website
www.kimmyfit.idlife.com
Don't make excuses. Make it F.I.T.!

--*Kimmy*

Booking Information

Kimmy Ross conducts live and virtual presentations on health, wellness and fitness for individuals, families, groups, churches, and organizations throughout the year.

To book an event:

Kimmy F.I.T. Fitness, LLC
11601 Shadow Creek Parkway #111, #136
Pearland, TX 77584

Voice Mail: 281-671-4540
www.kimmyfitfitness.com
Join my email list.

Email:
kimmyfitfitness@gmail.com
I invite your comments.
Twitter @Blazze02

Made in the USA
Lexington, KY
22 September 2017